MW01249227

Bodybuilding for Women

How to Build a Lean, Strong, and Fit Body by Home Workout

Kimberly Ward

Table of Contents

Introduction..1

CHAPTER ONE

The Benefits of Bodybuilding for Women 2

CHAPTER TWO

Bodybuilding Exercises at Home....................................5

   Warm-up Lifts: Bodybuilding Exercises at Home 5
      Cardio...5
      Dynamic Stretching 6
      Balance 10
   Upper Body Workouts 15
      Arms..16
      Chest 19
      Shoulders 21
      Back 22
   Abdominal and Core Workouts 25
      Abdominal..25
      Core 29
      Glute 32
   Lower Body Workouts 34
   Sample 7-Day Training Plan 41
   Bodybuilding Exercises at Home: Variety 47

CHAPTER THREE

Bodybuilding Nutrition 48

   Bodybuilding Nutrition: Focus on Protein 48
      Protein Shakes and Bars..................................50
   Bodybuilding Nutrition: Macros..................................51

What to Eat 52
The Vegetarian/Vegan Bodybuilder 53
Pre and Post-Workout Nutrition 54

CHAPTER FOUR

Bodybuilding Tips for Beginners **56**

Conclusion **60**

Introduction

Bodybuilding and weight lifting seem, to most people, like an inherently male pursuit. However, there are numerous benefits of bodybuilding for women. If you've been thinking about building up your body, improving your fitness level overall, or just becoming stronger—consider bodybuilding. You have a lot more than muscle to gain. Bodybuilding can promote weight loss, specifically the loss of fat. It also increases your strength, speed, and overall athletic performance. There are also health benefits; you'll decrease your risk for osteoporosis and increase blood and oxygen flow to all your major organs, including your brain.

With this guide, you will have at your fingertips everything you need to make the most of your bodybuilding experience, whether you are starting from scratch or need a handy-dandy reference to flip through if you get stuck.

Get ready, take a deep breath, and go!

CHAPTER ONE

The Benefits of Bodybuilding for Women

Even a beginner's bodybuilding routine will burn calories and fat. When you lift weights, you put your body through a series of resistance training moves to build muscle. This type of training not only replaces fat with muscle it also increases your metabolism. When your resting metabolism increases, your body begins to burn calories throughout the day and night, even at rest. This is a huge help when it comes to losing weight. Gaining muscle means burning extra calories and chiseling away at the fat deposits that have been plaguing you through other workout routines. Bodybuilding will leave you leaner and stronger.

In addition to weight loss, there are quite a few benefits of bodybuilding that sometimes go overlooked.

1. **More energy.** You'll be able to lift heavier weights or feel less tired after a particularly strenuous exercise session. Not just for exercise, but you'll also notice that you need less sleep to feel the full effect, and if you tend to catch an energy dip at 2 PM, you'll remedy this minor annoyance as well, allowing you to perform your best at work. Win, win.

2. **Sport training.** If you are currently involved in a sport such as swimming, tennis, or recreational team sports like softball or basketball, bodybuilding can help you improve your athletic performance. If you're not a natural athlete but want to look and feel like one, bodybuilding will nudge you closer to those goals.

3. **Self-esteem.** Your body will change as soon as you start lifting weights. The muscle tone will improve, you'll be faster and more flexible, and your overall physical presence will be more attractive and healthier. You'll feel a surge of confidence as well.

4. **Better health.** Lifting weights is good for your mind and body. Women are more susceptible to osteoporosis than men, and bodybuilding can help you minimize your risk. That's because your bone mineral density improves with weight lifting. You'll make both your muscles and your bones stronger and denser. The stronger connective tissue that you develop will also offset any risk of arthritis or joint swelling. Other risks go down when you're building your body with weights and resistance training, including the risk of heart disease and diabetes.

5. **Stress release.** Nothing beats a good weight lifting session, especially if you are stressed out. Physical exertion triggers the release of endorphins in the brain. Women bodybuilders are less likely to feel depressed. Lifting weights can also lift your mood.

The benefits of bodybuilding for women are outstanding, and if you haven't yet felt inspired to start lifting weights, you should seriously consider it. Try the home workouts in this book, and it won't be long before you begin to look and feel better.

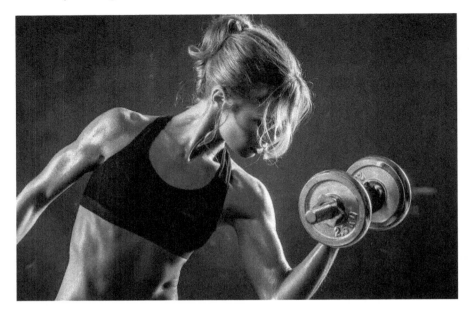

CHAPTER TWO

Bodybuilding Exercises at Home

While many bodybuilders enjoy going to a gym to work out, as a beginner, you may feel more comfortable at home. There are a lot of excellent weight lifting exercises you can get done in the privacy of your own home, and you don't need expensive equipment or a custom-made gym. Try these bodybuilding exercises at home to get an idea of how to move and lift to get stronger.

Warm-up Lifts: Bodybuilding Exercises at Home

Warming up is important when you're beginning a bodybuilding program because it signals to your body and mind that some physical activity is about to begin. These are some simple ways to get yourself ready for more intense exercise.

Cardio

Start with about 15 to 20 minutes of cardio warming up. This will elevate your heart rate, jumpstart your metabolism and get your muscles warm and loose. There are several options for the cardio component of your warm-up, and you should choose the one that is most appealing to you. A brisk 10-minute walk will do the trick, or you can jog or even sprint if you want to pick up the pace. Take a bike ride, do some jumping jacks, a little Zumba, or aerobics. The goal is to get your body moving and elevate your heart rate so you can move into the substance of your weight training workout.

Dynamic Stretching

A little flexibility will go a long way. As you build your body, you'll find that you're able to move better, and your body will feel more flexible. Stretching before and after your workouts will increase your flexibility and move you toward your strength goals.

Toe Touch

Start with some basic Toe Touches. Stand with your feet together and bend over slowly at the waist, with your arms stretched over your head. You'll feel a pull at the back of your legs but continue to lower yourself down towards the floor. Try to touch your fingertips to your toes. If you can't get that far the first time, that's alright. You'll get closer and closer the more you work at it. After a few seconds, raise yourself back up to a standing position. Do this five times.

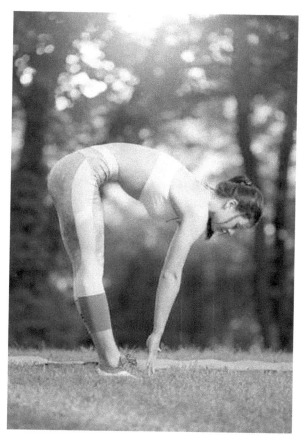

Quad Stretch

1. Remain standing from the previous position, inhale and exhale.

2. Keep your core tight as you lift your right foot behind you, gripping the ankle.

3. Stretch your quads and hold for 30 seconds per side.

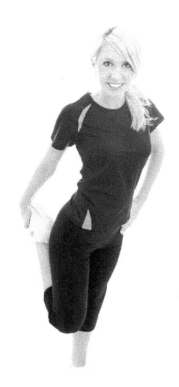

Linear Marches and Skips

Next, move into Linear Marches and Skips. The march is a simple movement where you raise your knee to the waist level and then return your foot to the floor. Repeat with the other foot. March three times across your room, going back and forth. Then, move it into a skip, where you jump while raising your knee and taking steps. Skip three times across your room, making sure that you raise your knees to your waist.

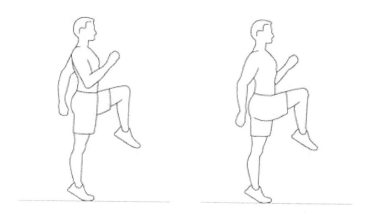

Arms Circle

The upper body needs to warm up next. Stand with your feet shoulder-width apart and complete some Arms Circles. Start with your hands by your sides, lift both arms together, and swing them in a complete circle. Do 1 set of 10 swings moving forward and 1 set of 10 swings going backward.

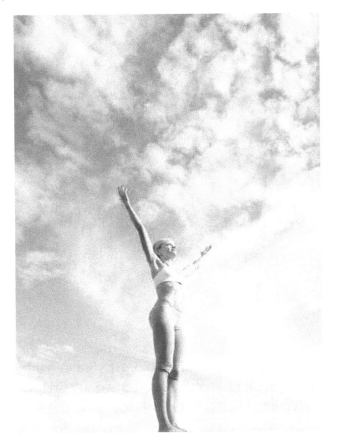

Balance

Balance is a major part of bodybuilding, and an element of your warm-up should include learning how to balance your body weight and stay focused.

Running in Place

Stand with your feet together and your arms by your side. Lift your left leg while lifting your right arm and bring them both back to the starting position. Switch, lifting the right leg and the left arm. Do 10 reps.

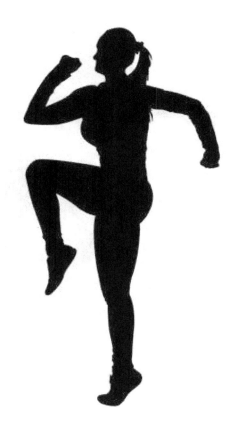

Duck Walk

Squat with your back straight and start walking slowly, never extending into a standing position but remaining in a squat with your back straight. Walk this way across your room 3 times.

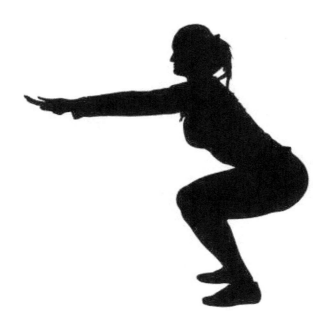

Yoga Tree Pose
Bring a bit of yoga.

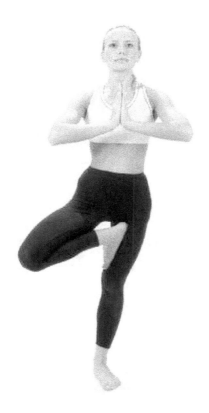

1. Stand straight and tall, arms at your side.

2. Keeping your hips forward, shift weight to your left leg and place the bottom of your foot inside your left thigh.

3. Balance yourself, then bring your hands in front of you, palms together in a prayer position.

4. Breath easily and reach arms up over your shoulders, palms separated and facing each other, holding for 30 seconds.

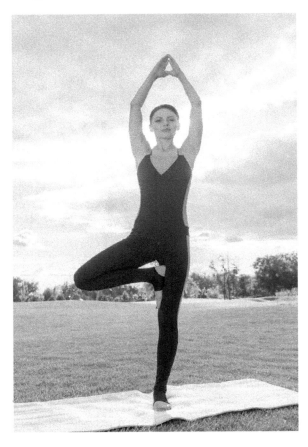

5. Lower arms and repeat with the opposite side.

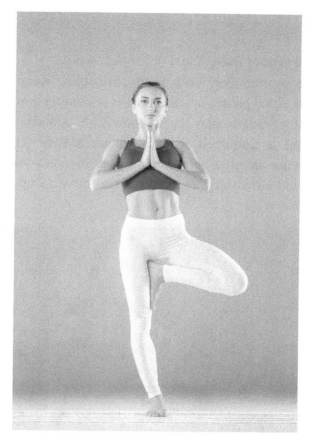

7. Repeat 5 times, alternating between left and right side.

Upper Body Workouts

When it's time to build your upper body, you want to focus on your arms, chest, shoulders, and back. These exercises are basic enough for beginners to master, but they'll also take you a long way towards a stronger top half.

Arms

Dumbbell Alternate Bicep Curl (12 reps/2 sets)

Either seated or standing, keep your core tight. Keep both arms down at your side, palms up. Start with a dumbbell weight that's comfortable for you. It may be 3 pounds, 5 pounds, or even 10 pounds. Using a dumbbell in each hand, slowly lift the right dumbbell to your shoulder, contracting your bicep as you lift. Hold the position and slowly lower the dumbbell down. Repeat with the other arm.

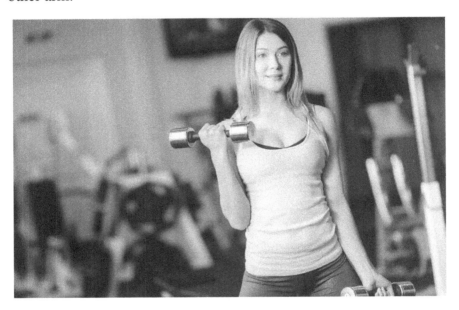

Concentration Curl (12 reps/3 sets)

Do this exercise on a chair or a bench. Flatten your back and put one hand on the chair seat or the bench. Use the other hand to grasp the dumbbell and allow your arm to hang straight at your side. Bend and lift your arm until your elbow is parallel with the side of your body. Hold for a second and straighten the arm again. Repeat with the other arm.

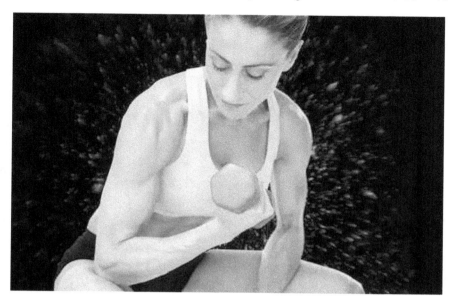

Bent-over Row (15 reps/4 sets)

On a bench, couch, or chair, support one knee and one hand on the bench. Keep one leg straight next to it on the floor. In your free hand, hold a dumbbell firmly. Curl the weight to your shoulder and release. Repeat with the other arm.

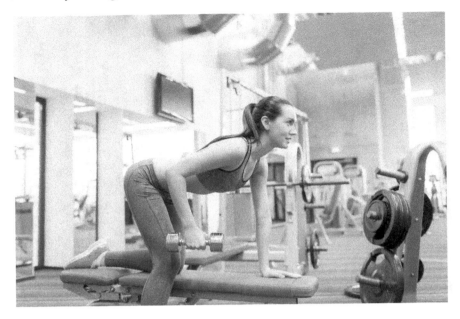

Resistance Pull

Use a resistance stretch band for 3 sets of 12 weight pulls. Step on the stretch band and grasp the ends in each hand. Hold your arms straight and bend them to curl up the same way you did with the dumbbells.

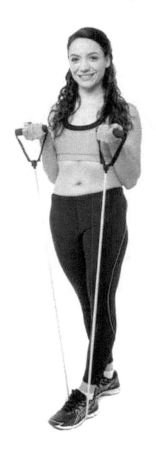

Chest

Chest Press (15 reps/3 sets)

This move can be done on the floor, but it is advised that you use a bench or similar surface. Lay on the bench (feet on either side on the floor and core tight) and hold dumbbells in each hand at a ninety-degree angle with palms towards your toes. Keep your elbows pointed out, and move the dumbbells close together at the top of your extension. Slowly release back to the starting position.

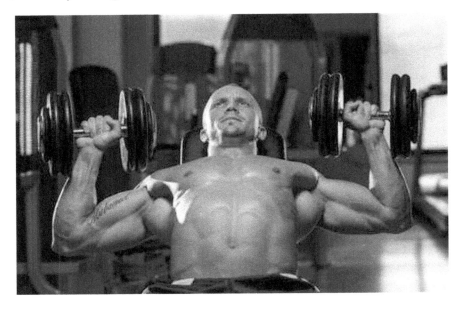

Dumbbell Fly (12 reps/2 sets)
Similar to the chest press, lay on the bench and keep your core tight. Hold dumbbells in each hand above the chest with elbows bent slightly. Lower the dumbbells to the sides until you feel chest muscles are stretched. Bring dumbbells together in front of your chest.

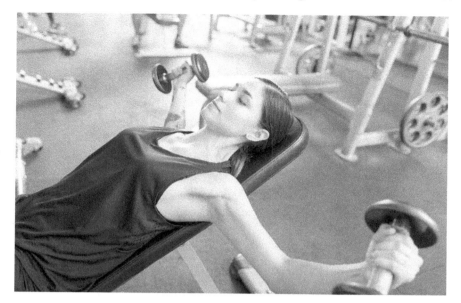

Shoulders

Shoulder Extension (12 reps/3 sets)
Stand with your legs shoulder-width apart and the dumbbells in your hands. Bend your arms, so the weights are right at your shoulders. Push them up into the air and past your head until your arms are almost straight. Slowly lower them back down to your shoulders.

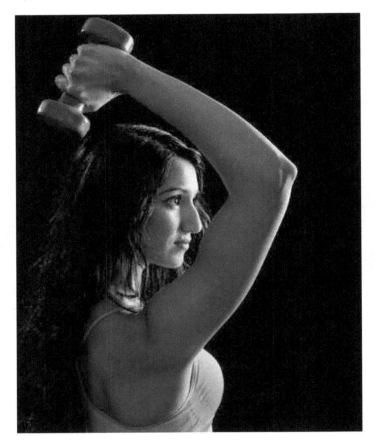

Back

Push-up (10 reps/3 sets)
Kneel on the floor and put your palms flat on the ground in front of you, shoulder-width apart. Keeping your back straight, lower your upper body towards the ground while staying on your knees. Once you nearly touch your chin to the floor, push yourself back up. As you get stronger, come off your knees and do traditional push-ups where your knees do not touch the ground.

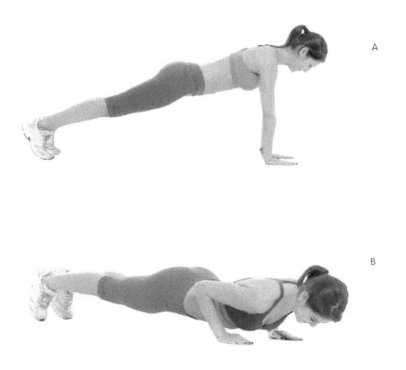

A

B

Pull-up (10 reps/2 sets)

If you have a strong structure or support in your house to use, this exercise is great for giving you that strong back as well as working the shoulders and biceps as stabilizing muscles. It might be a challenge if you are doing it for the first time, but your repetitions will increase as you get the hang of it.

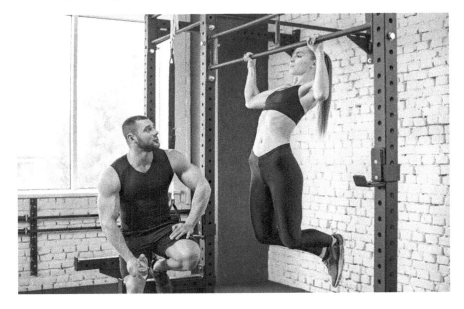

Position your hands about two inches wider than shoulder-width with your palms facing forward. Pull your body up slowly until your chin is at the same level as your hands, then slowly lower your body. You can bend your knees for improved stability.

Bench Dip/Triceps Dip (12 rep/2 sets)

You can use a sturdy chair or a bench for this move. As if you are sitting on air, place your hands on the bench behind you, fingers facing the same direction as your feet. Keep your knees together as you slowly lower yourself down. Hold the movement a few seconds before pushing up again.

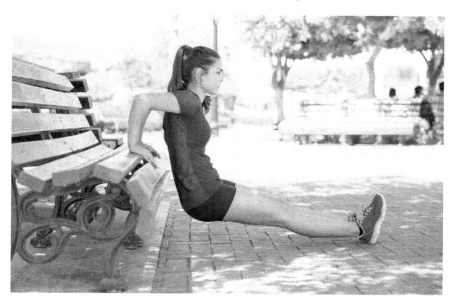

Abdominal and Core Workouts

You cannot build your body successfully without a strong core. The core includes your abs, your glutes, as well as the lower back. These exercises will give you the foundational strength to increase your bodybuilding results.

Abdominal

Frog Sit-up (10 reps/3 sets)
On your back, pull your knees up and let the bottoms of your feet touch. Keep your core muscles tight, and place your hands behind your head (lightly and without pulling). Keeping your legs in place, sit up with your upper body and lower back down flat.

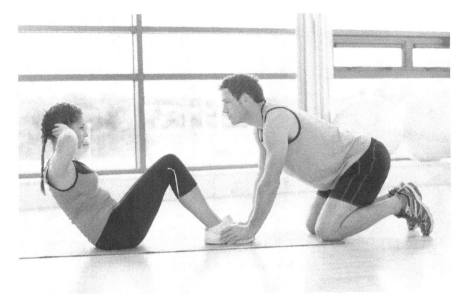

Hip Lift (10 reps/3 sets)
Lay on the floor with your legs lifted straight, so you're staring at your toes. Flex your feet and place your arms on the ground, at your sides. Without rocking or propelling your body, lift your hips a few inches off the ground, sending your feet towards the ceiling. Lower the hips again until your lower back is on the floor.

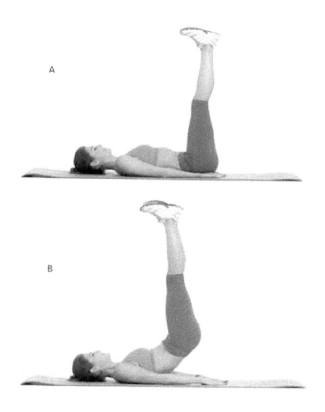

V-Up (10 reps/3 sets)

Lay on your back with your legs stretched out straight on the floor and your arms at your sides. Lift your head and shoulders at the same time you lift your legs until you reach a V position. Your arms should come up with your legs, so they are also off the ground. Lower yourself back down to the floor.

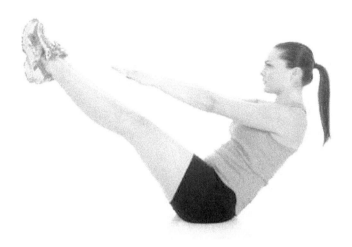

Reverse Crunch (10 reps/3 sets)

On your back, keep your legs together and bend your knees (keeping your feet flat on the floor). Place your arms flat on the floor by your side. Lift your lower body (legs still together) over your head, keeping your core tight and pressing against the floor with your arms for stability.

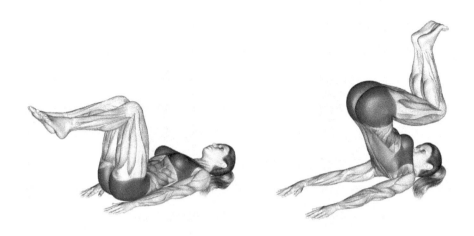

Core

Dumbbell Side Bend (8 reps/3 sets)

The key to this exercise is to keep your back straight and bend only at the waist. Stand with your feet shoulder-width apart, one dumbbell in your right hand. Keep your core tight, and bend to the right as far as possible. Return to the starting position and bend to the left as far as possible before returning to the starting position. Change the dumbbell to your left hand and repeat.

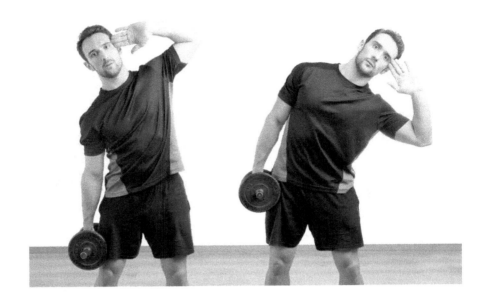

Downward Dog Kick (10 reps/3 sets)

Get on all fours and press your hips up and back, so you are in an inverted V shape. Lift your right leg and kick it behind you, keeping it straight. Do 10, and then switch to the left leg for 10.

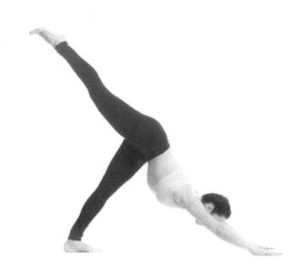

Plank

Hold a plank 3 times for at least 10 seconds. Lay on your stomach, with your toes curled under your feet, your elbows bent, and your hands flat on the floor. Push yourself up into the plank position so your arms are almost straight (don't lock the elbows) and your back is flat. You can also hold this position with your elbows on the floor, but many people find it more difficult.

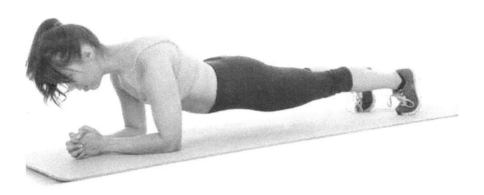

Glute

Hip Thrust (15 reps/3 sets)
Lying on your back, place your feet shoulder-width apart (feet in firm contact with the ground). Place your hands flat on the floor next to your body. Keep your core tight and thrust your hips into the air. Keep the movement slow and controlled. Squeeze your buttocks at the top of the movement and hold for a few seconds before releasing. You can balance weights on your pelvis for added resistance.

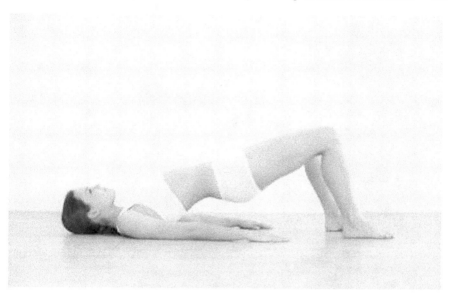

Leg Kick (10 reps/3 sets)

Get on all fours with your hands and knees shoulder-width apart. Extend your right leg, so it's straight and lift it as high as you can behind you. Bend the knee and bring it back without letting it touch the floor. Kick again. Kick the left leg after the right.

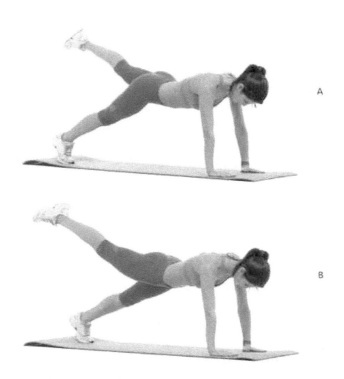

Lower Body Workouts

When focusing on your lower body, you want to improve the strength in your thighs, hamstrings, hips, and quadriceps. These exercises will promote muscle growth, balance, and range of motion.

Squat (12 reps/3 sets)
Standing with your feet shoulder-width apart and your hands extended in front of you. Bend your knees and slowly lower yourself towards the ground, lowering your torso and keeping your back

straight. Go as low as you can while maintaining the ability to press yourself back up to a standing position.

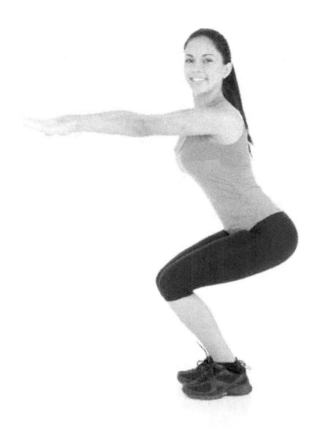

Squat with Weight (10 reps/3 sets)
Hold a kettlebell or a dumbbell with both hands in front of you. As you squat, bend your arms and raise the weight to your chest. Lower the weight as you straighten out of the squat.

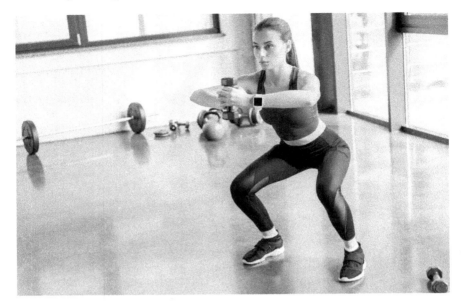

Lunge (10 reps/3 sets)

Stand with your feet together and take one step, bending both legs so that your leading leg bends to almost 90 degrees and your back knee nearly touches the floor. Keep your back straight. Slowly come up out of the movement and step back, so your feet are back together. Alternate the right and left legs.

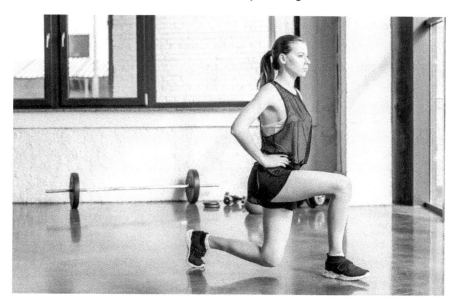

Lunge with Weight (10 reps/3 sets)
Complete your lunges while holding a dumbbell in each hand.

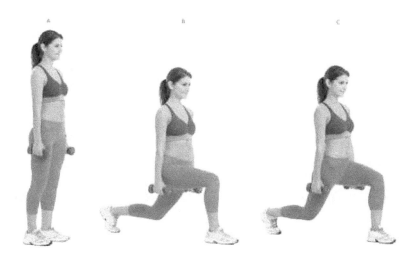

Hip Extender (10 reps/3 sets)

Stand with legs together, holding the back of a chair or a barre for support. Swing your right leg back behind you, keeping your back straight and the left leg straight. Lower it back to the ground. After doing 10 on your right side, switch to the left leg.

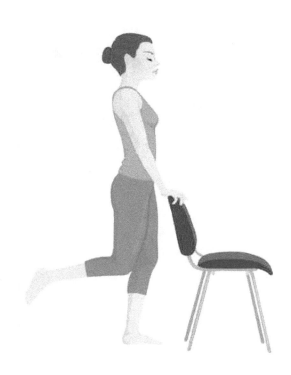

Toe Raise (15 reps/3 sets)

Stand with your legs together, holding the back of a chair for support. Lift yourself up onto your toes, feeling your muscles tighten in your calves. Lower yourself back to the ground. Don't rest for more than a second before lifting yourself up onto your toes again.

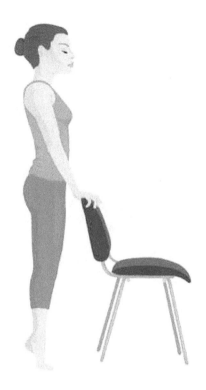

Jumping Jacks (30 reps/3 sets)

Most of us know what jumping jacks are and have done it when we were kids. This exercise is great for working the glutes, hip flexors, and quads. It also hits the abs, calves, hamstrings, and shoulders as stabilizing muscles.

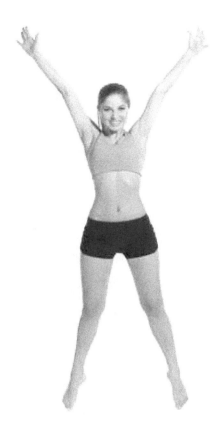

It is a great exercise that builds strength as well as endurance at the same time. This is a great finisher for your daily workout.

Sample 7-Day Training Plan

Now that you understand what kinds of workouts you can incorporate with bodybuilding exercises at home, you need to think about your fitness routine for full weeks at a time. When you're planning what to do, make sure you're focusing on all areas of strength training. It's also important to rest, so your body and your muscles can recover. Here's a sample 7-Day plan that makes an excellent template for beginning bodybuilders.

Day 1 − Lower Body

1. Start with a 10-minute warm-up. Walk briskly around your neighborhood or on your treadmill if you have one at home. Since it's a lower-body workout day, spend another 5 minutes warming up those legs and hips. Do 3 sets of marches and 3 sets of skips.

2. Do 3 sets of 12 squats.

3. Do 3 sets of 10 lunge steps.

4. Do 3 sets of 10 Hip Thrusts.

5. Do 3 sets of 10 Hip Extenders for each leg.

6. Do the **Warrior Pose**. This is a yoga pose that strengthens the lower back and the legs. Move your right foot at least three or four feet in front of you, with the toe pointing to the front. Turn your left leg as needed to stretch it and keep your balance. Lift your arms over your head and stare at your palms, allowing the front leg to support most of your weight. Hold for at least 15 seconds, then switch, so the left leg is in front.

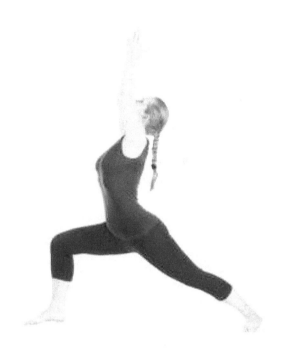

Day 2 – Upper Body

1. Start with a 10-minute warm-up. Walk or jog. Spend 5 more minutes warming up your arms with 3 sets of 10 arm circles.

2. Do 2 sets of 10 pull-ups.

3. Do 3 sets of 12 resistance pulls with a stretch band.

4. Do 3 sets of 12 **Arm Raises**. Hold a dumbbell in each hand and let your arms hang straight at your sides. Lift your arms to about shoulder height. Bring them slowly back down until they're at rest. Lift them again. Keep your arms straight.

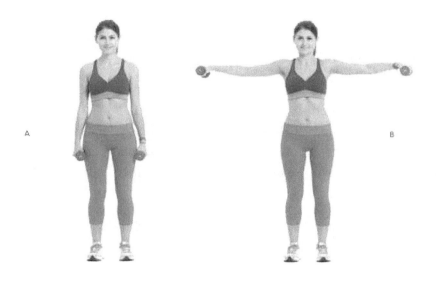

5. Do 3 sets of 10 push-ups.

Day 3 – Rest

On your rest day, continue to pay attention to your nutrition. Get some informal physical activity in if you can. Take a walk, go for a swim, or run after your kids at the park.

To maximize the impact of bodybuilding workouts, it is important to point out that muscle growth does not occur when you are working out. Instead, the repair and growth of muscles occur after the workout, when you are resting. For this reason, eating a nutritious diet and having a good rest are critical for bodybuilding.

Day 4 – Core

1. Warm up with 10 minutes of jumping jacks or jumping rope. You can also run in place or walk briskly. Spend another 5 minutes

doing neck rolls, where you first nod your head yes and then roll it in complete circles.

2. Do 3 sets of 10 shoulder shrugs. Stand with your feet together and lift your shoulders towards your ears. Slowly lower them.

3. Hold a plank for at least 10 seconds.

4. Do 3 sets of 10 V-Ups.

5. Hold another plank for at least 10 seconds.

6. Do 3 sets of 15 **Side Bends**. Stand with your feet shoulder-width apart. Bend to one side, lifting the opposite arm over your head. Come back to the center and bend the other way, lifting your other arm over your head.

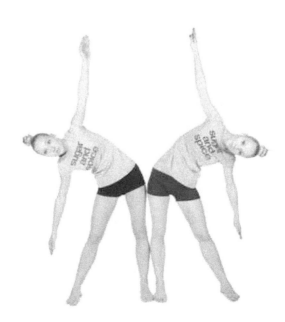

7. Do 3 sets of 10 Frog Sit-ups.

Day 5 – Lower Body

1. Warm up with a brisk 10-minute walk or a jog. Spend 5 more minutes doing marches and skips.

2. Do 3 sets of 12 **Chair Squats**. This is the same movement as a regular squat, but you'll do it standing in front of a chair. Lower yourself until you just reach the chair, and then push yourself back up.

3. Do 3 sets of 15 Toe Raises.

4. Do 3 sets of 12 **Side Leg Lifts**. Lay on the floor on your right side. Support your upper body on your elbow and stretch your legs out. Keeping your right leg on the floor, lift your left leg as high as it will go and lower it. Switch and do the other side as well.

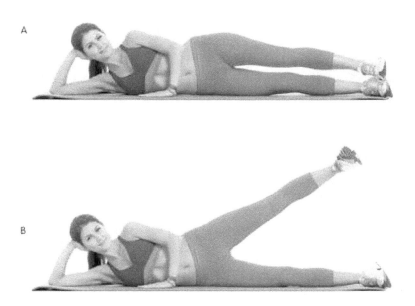

5. Do 3 sets of 10 **Side Lunges**. Stand with your feet together and your hands on your hips. Take a large step to the right side, lunging as deep as you can without falling. Push yourself back to the center position. Alternate to the left side.

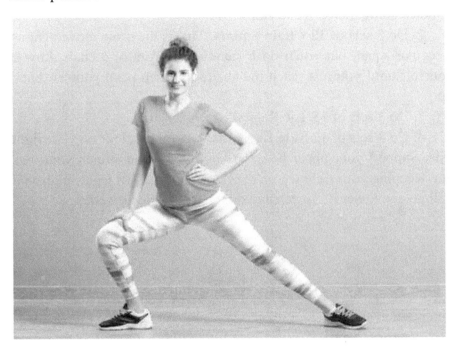

Day 6 − Rest
You may be feeling sore, especially after another lower body workout day. Allow your body to rest, and take a leisurely walk so you can stretch out those recovering muscles.

Day 7 − Core and Upper Body
1. Warm up with a 10-minute walk or jog. Spend 5 minutes doing neck rolls, shoulder rolls, and toe raises.

2. Hold a plank for at least 10 seconds.
3. Do 3 sets of 10 V-Ups
4. Do 3 sets of 15 Hip Thrusts.
5. Do 3 sets of 10 Hip Lifts.
6. Do 3 sets of 10 push-ups.

Bodybuilding Exercises at Home: Variety

It's important not to get bored. As your strength and endurance improve, you'll find that the repetitions seem easier, and you can take on more weight when you're using dumbbells, kettlebells, or other weights. You always want to be looking for new exercises to incorporate into your bodybuilding plan. The exercises in this book are meant to be good for beginners so you can start to understand how your body feels physically and what kind of capacity you have for growth. If you begin to feel bored or the routines get monotonous, try different exercises and learn other ways to increase your strength and build your body. Remember that while your focus isn't on cardio but strength training, there's still a place for some light cardio exercises. It's good for your heart, legs, and overall physical fitness.

These bodybuilding exercises can be done at home. When you're ready to progress to some weight lifting machines, you can join a gym to support your efforts. For now, get to know these simple exercises to build an excellent foundation for your training program. Some people find they are more successful when they work out with a friend. If you decide to do this, go over the plan and the program to ensure that you're on track according to your current abilities and plans for growth.

CHAPTER THREE

Bodybuilding Nutrition

When you decide to launch a bodybuilding routine, it's important to pay attention to your nutrition. What you eat will fuel your body and provide you with the nutrients that are necessary to build and maintain muscle. Instead of placing yourself on a strict diet and limiting the foods and calories you eat, it's important to eat enough to help you reach a peak physical performance. Your bodybuilding nutrition should focus on protein, which is essential to getting stronger and keeping your metabolism in a fat-burning and muscle-growing mode.

Bodybuilding Nutrition: Focus on Protein

Protein repairs and rebuilds just about anything in the body but is incredibly important for creating new muscle and repairing muscle damage. Whenever you exercise or place strain on your muscles, it causes micro tears in the muscle fiber itself. Protein repairs and builds on this tear, causing the muscle to become stronger and bigger. The more protein you get, the faster and more efficient this process is. When you begin a bodybuilding schedule, you need to increase your protein intake because you're not only sustaining a healthy and strong body; you're building one.

If you plan on combining your bodybuilding with a diet such as Keto, you definitely need to be aware that if you are not getting enough protein, you will not see as much improvement as you would want to.

The best protein sources come directly from foods. You can eat eggs, fish, and lean meats such as chicken, turkey, beef, and pork. Protein can also be found in nuts and seeds, as well as legumes, beans, and tofu. Some people supplement their diets with protein shakes, powders, and bars. This is a good way to give yourself an energy boost and add valuable protein ingredients to your diet. However, you should try to eat as much natural protein as you can so you don't get hungry. Start your day with a plate of eggs; a good breakfast packed with protein will give you a great base to build, and you'll have the energy you need to get through your workouts and your day.

Consuming protein as part of your bodybuilding nutrition helps you in other ways. You'll feel fuller, so you won't have to worry about snacking on unhealthy foods during the day. The protein will help you burn fat more effectively as well because it has a positive impact on your metabolism. Your body will convert the protein into glucose, which means you'll have more energy. Diets higher in protein and lower in carbohydrates have also been proven to assist with weight loss and better heart health.

Many protein sources also come with fats. Don't worry too much about that. Your body also needs the fat, especially as you're building muscle. As long as you're eating healthy fats, such as oils, fish, and nuts, you're serving your body well.

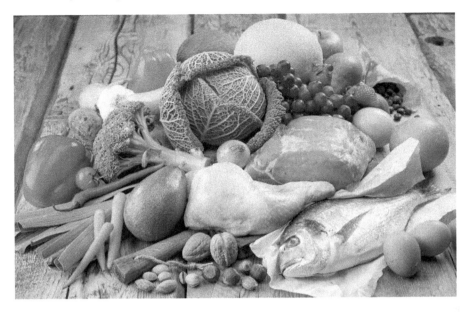

Protein Shakes and Bars

Not only are protein shakes super easy to throw together, but they also give you a boost to your protein requirements for the day, allowing you to focus on your workouts and stress less about not getting enough protein.

Whey protein is a popular choice. It is often incorporated into the diet twice a day and is more readily absorbed by the system than traditional forms of protein.

When you start looking at protein shakes and other supplements, be careful and read the label. A good protein shake has a base of 70%–90% protein. Many items you find on the shelves these days tend to be closer to 60% and lower, having been bulked up with carbs and sugars.

There are also great vegan and vegetarian-friendly protein powders available at health stores. Look for plant-based powders or powders formed around pea and nut flours (as well as milk).

If you opt for the protein bar, you can look at the ready-made snacks in the health food aisles. Be sure to read the labels—sugar comes in many different forms.

Bodybuilding Nutrition: Macros

Macronutrients, or macros, are what make up any kind of food or drink: protein, fat, and carbohydrates. Two more components are as important but do not quite classify as macronutrients: water and fiber. We have talked about protein in the previous section. We will now discuss the roles of other macros in bodybuilding.

Carbohydrates
Carbohydrates provide the body with fuel. It is the primary source of fuel and gets broken down into glucose. Your body stores glucose as glycogen in the cells. When you exercise, it is the first fuel that will be burned for energy. Once the glycogen stores are depleted, your body will turn to fat and protein in muscles to burn as fuel.

Fat
Fat helps lubricate joints, skin, and hair. It also creates a safety barrier around your organs to protect them. If you feel like your joints are a little sore and have been hitting your protein macros consistently, you may need to include a little more fat into your diet.

Water
Water hydrates. The more protein you consume, the more water you will need to drink. The process of breaking down protein in the body tends to use a ton more water. Water binds to muscles as well. Water hydrates the skin and often sits as a sort of barrier beneath the skin. It is responsible for nearly all the processes in the body.

Water also carries micronutrients around the body in the bloodstream. Micronutrients are the smaller building blocks such as vitamins and minerals that your body utilizes for essential functions in the body.

Fiber
Fiber keeps things running smoothly. Too much protein will cause unpleasant experiences in the bathroom and is often the biggest cause of diarrhea (non-illness related, of course). Fiber improves gut health and reduces the risk of heart disease. Fiber doesn't get absorbed by the body but gets discarded after it has served its purpose.

What to Eat

Most successful bodybuilders follow a diet that is high in protein and good carbohydrates. Processed foods high in sugar, added fats, and salt will only slow you down and contribute to weight gain. If you're going to gain weight while bodybuilding, you want to make sure that you're gaining lean, healthy muscle and not fat. The way to do that is by putting together a diet that is balanced, nutritious, and compatible with a bodybuilding routine.

   1. **Lean meat**: chicken is your new best friend. Build meals around chicken, turkey, and lean beef.
   2. **Cold water fish**: a little higher in fat but has higher omega 3 fatty acids that aid muscle growth. High in protein, tuna and salmon are great alternatives to chicken.
   3. **Sweet potato**: it is a good source of carbohydrates and fiber. While it has a bit more sugar than white potatoes, it is evened out by having more fiber. It will keep you fuller for longer.
   4. **Green vegetables**: broccoli and spinach. If you don't have a taste for these, it's time to start growing attached. These two veggies have all the vitamins and minerals your body needs (iron, for one, is important for adequate, healthy blood flow). Vegetables are

carbohydrates, but when balanced with the amount of fiber, the carb levels are low enough that you can eat enough of these to feel full without the guilt. Learn to love your green veggies.

5. **Egg whites**: yes, it tastes like it's missing something. However, it is also one of the purest forms of protein. With no carbohydrates and very little fat, the balance of protein to calories is astounding.

6. **Beans and legumes**: a little explosion of energy. Things like chickpeas (garbanzo beans) and lentils are high in protein and fiber. Tread carefully though, as they do contain quite a bit of carbs.

Remember that even though you are trying to "put on weight, " it needs to happen gradually and in a healthy manner. Start with focusing on your protein. Then add in the other macros. Pay attention to what your body needs and take it from there. If you feel depleted too often and too early during or before workouts, look at what you eat.

- 30–35% protein
- 55–60% carbs
- 15–20% fat

Beware of fad diets. While losing weight might be one of your fitness goals, you do not want to limit your caloric intake too dramatically. If you do that, your body won't be able to increase in strength and muscle. Instead of counting calories, pay attention to the types of food you choose. What you eat will matter much more than how many calories or fat grams are present.

The Vegetarian/Vegan Bodybuilder

Bodybuilding as a vegetarian or vegan is slightly more challenging than when you have few to no dietary restrictions. The bulk of protein for bodybuilders comes from eating chicken. However, you can carefully adapt your diet to plant-based proteins.

There are quite a variety of plant-based proteins to choose from when designing your high-protein diet. Unlike the general populace of bodybuilders, you will need to change the source of your protein frequently to benefit in the same way.

Not all proteins are created equal, nor do they all contain the same amino acids that your body requires to function optimally as it builds up muscle. These plant-based proteins contain varying levels of the essential amino acids and, therefore, should be combined and varied as much as possible. Be aware of the carb content in certain plant-based sources as well.

Listed below are a few plant-based proteins that you should be incorporating into your diet in order to ensure a well-rounded selection of amino acids for optimum health:

- Quinoa
- Soybeans and other soy products (tofu and edamame)
- Buckwheat
- Brown and wild rice
- Legumes (chickpeas, green peas, and lentils)
- Seitan
- Nutritional yeast
- Spirulina supplements
- Chia seeds and nuts
- Eggs and milk for the ovo-lacto vegetarians

Pre and Post-Workout Nutrition

What you eat before and after your bodybuilding workouts will have a major impact on how you perform. Before your workout, eat some protein with high-quality carbohydrates, so you have the energy you need to lift weights and build your body. If you like to work out in the morning, try scrambled eggs on top of a piece of high-fiber toast or whole-grain oats topped with nuts and fruit. If you hit the gym in the afternoon or evening, brown rice or pasta is good to eat about an hour before starting your bodybuilding.

After a workout, you need to have some protein, which will help your muscles recover. Have some grilled chicken or a piece of fish. If you aren't craving a full meal, try a protein shake or a protein bar to feed and repair your muscles. Make sure you stay hydrated and avoid foods high in the glycemic index. These will drain your energy and contribute to feeling tired during your bodybuilding workout. Empty carbohydrates from junk foods and sugars are not good to consume, especially before or after your workouts.

Your bodybuilding nutrition is essential but second to your workouts. The best way to build your body is through consistent and challenging weight lifting. You'll need to dedicate yourself to spending time with weights and increasing the amount of your exercise. When you combine that with the right foods, you will be impressed with the results you're able to achieve.

CHAPTER FOUR

Bodybuilding Tips for Beginners

Once you begin a bodybuilding routine, it's natural to be enthusiastic. However, pacing yourself is important. You don't want to overdo your early workouts and burn out, or put yourself at risk for injury. These are some bodybuilding tips for beginners that will help you devote your time and focus to the practice of bodybuilding without expecting unrealistic results from yourself.

1. Work at your own pace
You may work your way up to the competitive circuit, but when you're starting, there is no one to compete with except yourself. The goal is to work at your own pace and let yourself improve over time. There is no sense in comparing yourself to people who have been lifting weights for years or trying to outpace a workout partner who is doing some bodybuilding as well.

Stay focused on yourself and what you want to accomplish. Start slowly and with the number of workouts that you're comfortable with. If you lift weights seven days a week, for two hours a day, you'll probably end up disappointed, sore, and unable to continue. Set small, realistic goals. Maybe start with two days a week or a minimal amount of weight. Set a slower pace to begin, and see if you can build off that.

2. Increase intensity gradually
Once you find a comfortable and sustainable pace, increase your intensity gradually. Move from a 10-pound weight to 15-pound weight and keep adding more over time as your lifting becomes easier. Do the same thing with your repetitions. Start by lifting eight times, then 10 times, then 12 times, and then 15. You will learn to

figure out how you feel and how much weight your muscles can list. Going slowly will prevent injuries and keep you from becoming discouraged if you try to increase too much too fast. Trust your body and take your time. Bodybuilding isn't a race. It's a long-term fitness plan. Increase your weight every two weeks.

3. Focus on free weights

Depending on your gym, you might find yourself dazzled by fancy machines and complex contraptions. But remember that free weights are the best way to start a bodybuilding routine, and you can even use them at home. Barbells and dumbbells will help you build a solid foundation of lean muscle mass, and you can move to the machines later, when you're stronger and need a more complex challenge. Invest in some free weights in various sizes and weight levels so you can do some lifting regardless of where you are.

4. Take days off

Many beginners are so excited about their plans that they want to work out every day. However, your body needs rest, and your muscles will use your off days to recover and repair themselves in time for your next workout. Isolate the muscle groups so you can do legs one day and then chest and arms the next day. Try sticking to a routine of three or four days per week. This will give you enough of a schedule that you get accustomed to working out every other day, but your body won't get too sore, and you won't run the risk of injury.

5. Learn proper form

If you're not sure what you're supposed to be doing or how you're supposed to be lifting, partner up with someone who does or consider working with a personal trainer. As a beginner, if you learn bad techniques, you will have a hard time breaking those habits. This could mean that you have to stick with lower weight levels for a while; until you're able to capture and maintain the right form. It will be worth it for you as you progress, however.

6. Don't skip the warm-up
You may be tempted to do this because you're running short on time, or something has come up, and you can't dedicate the amount of time you normally would to your exercise program. Don't skip the warm-up, as you will increase the risk of injury.

7. Make safety a priority
Try to work out with a partner who can spot you, especially during big lifts. Wear a safety belt when you start lifting weight that is more than you've lifted before and don't be afraid to ask for help. Beginners have a lot to learn from experienced bodybuilders, and most people committed to this lifestyle are willing to offer tips and advice. Some bodybuilders need gloves to protect their hands. Take every safety precaution you can, and be careful when working out.

8. Watch your nutrition
As you know, what you eat has a major impact on how you lift. So stay away from junk food, eat a lot of protein, and make sure you are hydrated before, during, and after workouts. Don't limit your calories, and make sure you eat enough to support the amount of energy you need to put out during your weight lifting sessions.

9. Try compound moves
This means you need to focus on exercises that utilize more than one muscle group per movement. Keep it simple in the beginning. Don't overcomplicate your workout. Instead, do the basics. You should complete squats weekly, deadlifts, bench presses, and shoulder lifts. Focus on those basics, and then build off your momentum into other types of lifts that focus on the muscle groups you need to develop.

10. Stick to your program

Once you develop a routine, stick with it. Consistency will bring you greater results than anything else. As long as you manage to hit each muscle group every week and you feel like you've challenged yourself without overdoing it, you're getting a good workout in.

11. Take a holistic approach

Bodybuilding requires excellent overall health. Don't sabotage your plans by drinking, smoking, and doing drugs. Make sure you get enough sleep every night and learn how to manage your stress. If you want to build an outstanding body, it takes more than weight lifting. It takes a commitment to overall health.

These 11 bodybuilding tips for beginners can help you improve your chances of building a better body. Follow them and figure out what works best for you. It's going to increase your results and your rate of bodybuilding success.

Conclusion

Bodybuilding offers numerous benefits for women. It can be tailored to your daily schedule and fitness level. Start with small weights and a few repetitions, and you'll be surprised at how quickly you increase what you're able to do. Listen to what your body says. You do not need to push yourself to physical pain to see results.

You do, however, need the commitment that goes with it.

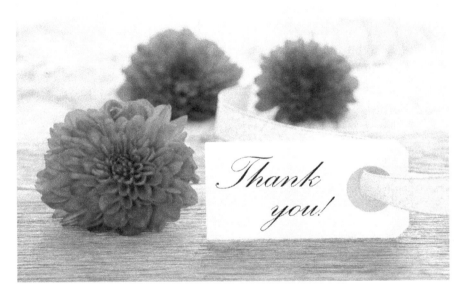

Finally, I want to thank you for reading my book. If you enjoyed the book, please share your thoughts and post a review on the book retailer's website. It would be greatly appreciated!

Best wishes,
Kimberly Ward